LOW SODIUM COOKBOOK FOR BEGINNERS

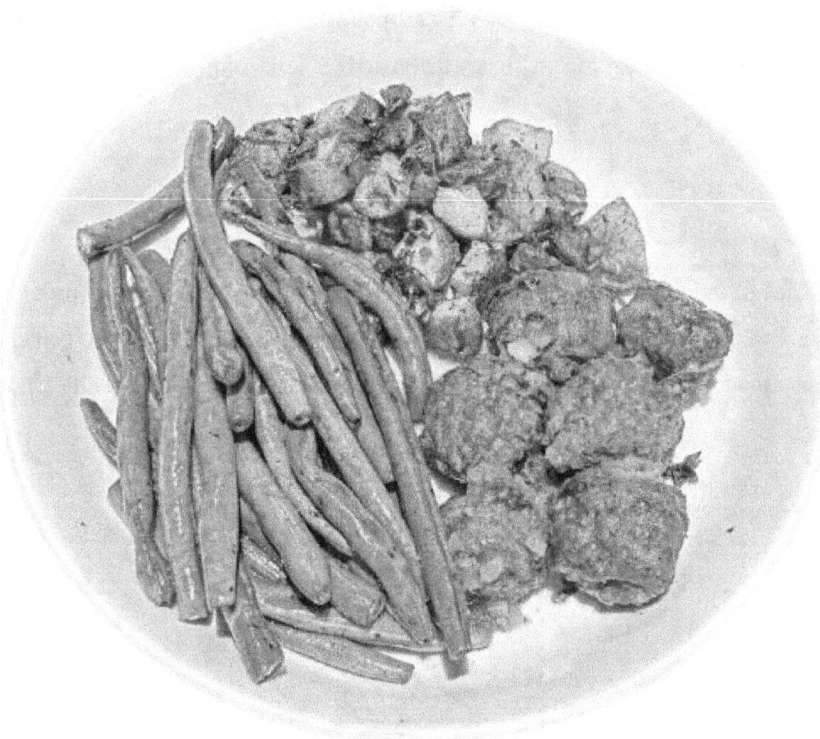

LORENE PEACHEY

TABLE OF CONTENTS

INTRODUCTION

Hello there, my fellow culinary adventurers! I'm Nutrionist Lorene Peachey, and today, I want to take you on a journey – a journey that started with a quest for flavour, health, and a dash of creativity in the kitchen. Welcome to my low sodium cookbook for beginners, a delightful collection of recipes that will transform your relationship with food and redefine the joy of healthy eating.

Let me share a little secret with you, a story that unfolded in the kitchen of someone I'd like to introduce you to – a vibrant soul named Maggie Whitman. Now, Maggie was on a mission. A mission that many of us embark upon at some point in our lives – the quest for a heart-healthy lifestyle. She had tried her hand at numerous cookbooks, each promising a path to flavour without the guilt, but alas, the results were far from satisfying.

One day, as Maggie navigated her way through culinary confusion, she stumbled upon my cookbook. With a sceptical glance, she decided to give it a whirl. Little did she know, this encounter would be a game-changer.

As she flipped through the pages, her eyes widened at the possibilities – Wholesome Main Courses, Satisfying Soups and Stews, Wholesome Snacks and Appetizers, and so much more. Intrigued, she decided to dive in. The first recipe she attempted was the Teriyaki Salmon with Brown Rice. The aroma filled her kitchen, and the Flavors danced on her palate. A revelation! This was the taste she had been searching for, a taste that screamed "healthy" without compromising on satisfaction.

Maggie's culinary escapade continued with each turn of the page. Eggplant and Chickpea Tagine, Baked Zucchini Chips, and the tantalizing Mushroom and Spinach Quiche with Oat Crust. The variety seemed endless, and Maggie was hooked. It wasn't just about low sodium; it was about savouring life, one delicious bite at a time.

Now, let's pause for a moment and reflect on something we all, at some point, ponder: What does it truly mean to Savor life? It's not just about the food on our plates; it's about the moments we create around them. It's about nourishing our bodies with love, embracing Flavors that elevate our spirits, and choosing a path that nurtures our well-being.

Consider this – what if every meal you savoured brought not just joy to your taste buds, but also a surge of vitality to your body? What if you could indulge in the richness of life without compromising on your health? These questions are not just food for thought; they are the essence of our journey.

So, why low sodium? The answer lies in the heartbeat of our bodies. High sodium intake, as many of us know, is often linked to a range of health issues. The consequence of unchecked sodium levels can be detrimental – elevated blood pressure, increased risk of heart disease, and a cascade of other concerns. It's not merely a culinary choice; it's a decision that impacts the very rhythm of our lives.

But fear not! The advantages of embracing a low sodium diet extend far beyond the avoidance of health pitfalls. It's about embracing a lifestyle that champions heart health, weight management, and overall well-being. And in this cookbook, my dear friend, you'll find not just recipes but a guide to a life well-lived.

Imagine the satisfaction of biting into a juicy Stuffed Bell Pepper Bite, the crunch of Baked Zucchini Chips echoing through your kitchen, or the comforting warmth of a Satisfying Soup on a chilly evening. These aren't just recipes; they are stories waiting to be written in the narrative of your health journey.

What sets this cookbook apart, you might ask? It's the simplicity, the variety, and the understanding that each meal is an opportunity to nourish both body and soul. These recipes aren't just low sodium; they are a celebration of culinary artistry tailored for beginners. Whether you're a kitchen novice or a seasoned chef, each page is an invitation to explore, experiment, and indulge.

As you embark on this adventure, consider the benefits – not just for your health but for the sheer joy of cooking. The aroma of herbs, the vibrant colours on your plate, and the knowledge that you're investing in your well-being – it's a symphony of experiences that extend far beyond the confines of your kitchen.

So, my dear friend, as you turn the pages of this cookbook, let the questions linger: What if every meal could be a celebration? What if your journey to a healthier you started with a single recipe? The answers are within these pages, waiting to be uncovered.

As you Savor each bite, let it be a reminder – a reminder that every choice we make in the kitchen is a step towards a more vibrant, healthier, and fulfilling life. It's a journey of self-discovery, a journey to savouring life – one heart-healthy recipe at a time.

So, are you ready to embark on this journey? Are you ready to redefine the way you think about low sodium cooking? Open this cookbook not just as a guide but as a companion on your culinary expedition. Let the recipes be the muse, the kitchen your canvas, and the Flavors your masterpiece.

As Nutrionist Lorene Peachey, I invite you to embrace the joy of cooking, the pleasure of savouring life, and the beauty of nourishing your body. Together, let's turn every meal into a celebration, every bite into a proclamation of well-being. Welcome to "Low Sodium Cookbook for Beginners." Your adventure begins now.

Contact the Author

Thank you for reading my book! I would love to hear from you, whether you have feedback, questions, or just want to share your thoughts. Your feedback means a lot to me and helps me improve as a writer.

Please don't hesitate to reach out to me through

lorenepeachey@gmail.com

I look forward to connecting with my readers and appreciate your support in this literary journey. Your thoughts and comments are valuable to me.

CHAPTER 1

UNDERSTANDING SODIUM AND ITS IMPACT

Sodium is an essential mineral that plays a crucial role in various bodily functions, including the regulation of blood pressure, fluid balance, and nerve function. However, excessive sodium intake can have detrimental effects on health, particularly on cardiovascular health. The primary source of sodium in the modern diet is often table salt (sodium chloride), but it is also found in many processed and packaged foods.

The Impact of Excessive Sodium Intake:

High Blood Pressure: Consuming too much sodium can lead to an increase in blood pressure. Elevated blood pressure is a major risk factor for heart disease, stroke, and other cardiovascular problems.

Fluid Retention: Sodium helps regulate fluid balance in the body. Excessive sodium can lead to water retention, causing bloating and swelling, particularly in the extremities.

Kidney Strain: The kidneys play a vital role in maintaining sodium balance in the body. High sodium intake can strain the kidneys, potentially leading to kidney problems over time.

Benefits of a Low Sodium Diet:

Heart Health: Reducing sodium intake is associated with lower blood pressure, reducing the risk of heart disease and stroke.

Kidney Function: A low sodium diet can ease the strain on the kidneys, promoting better kidney function and reducing the risk of kidney disease.

Fluid Balance: Maintaining a healthy sodium balance helps prevent fluid retention and reduces bloating.

Bone Health: High sodium intake is linked to increased calcium excretion in urine, which may contribute to bone loss. A low sodium diet can help preserve bone health.

Getting Started: Tips for Beginners

Read Labels: Be mindful of sodium content in packaged foods by reading nutrition labels. Choose low-sodium or sodium-free alternatives when possible.

Cook at Home: Home-cooked meals allow you to control the ingredients and salt content in your dishes. Use herbs, spices, and other flavorings to enhance taste without relying on excessive salt.

Choose Fresh Foods: Whole, fresh foods such as fruits, vegetables, lean meats, and whole grains generally contain lower levels of sodium compared to processed foods.

Limit Processed Foods: Processed and pre-packaged foods often contain high levels of sodium. Minimize your intake of canned soups, sauces, and snacks.

Gradual Reduction: If you're used to a high-sodium diet, consider gradually reducing salt in your meals. Your taste buds will adapt over time.

Hydration: Drinking plenty of water helps flush excess sodium from the body, supporting overall health.

CHAPTER 2

BASICS OF LOW SODIUM COOKING

Cooking with reduced sodium doesn't mean sacrificing flavor; it's about making conscious choices to promote a healthier lifestyle. Here are some essential principles to guide you in low sodium cooking:

Fresh Ingredients: Opt for fresh fruits, vegetables, lean meats, and whole grains. These whole foods are naturally lower in sodium compared to their processed counterparts.

Herbs and Spices: Use herbs and spices to enhance the flavor of your dishes. Experiment with a variety of seasonings such as garlic, onion, basil, oregano, thyme, and rosemary to add depth without relying on salt.

Citrus Juices: Citrus fruits like lemon and lime can add a zesty kick to your recipes. Squeeze fresh citrus juice onto salads, meats, or vegetables to brighten flavors.

Homemade Stocks: Prepare your own stocks and broths using fresh ingredients to control the sodium content. This allows you to enjoy the rich, savory taste of homemade soups and stews without excessive salt.

Reading Food Labels

Understanding food labels is crucial when adopting a low sodium diet. Here are tips for interpreting and making informed choices:

Check Sodium Content: Examine the sodium content per serving. Choose products labeled as "low sodium" or "no added salt."

Serving Size Awareness: Pay attention to the serving size specified on the label. The sodium content listed is often based on a single serving, so adjust accordingly if you consume more or less.

Look for Hidden Sodium: Ingredients like monosodium glutamate (MSG), sodium nitrate, and sodium benzoate can contribute to sodium intake. Be aware of these additives and choose products without them when possible.

Compare Brands: Similar products from different brands may have varying sodium levels. Compare labels to make the best choice for your low sodium needs.

Salt Alternatives and Substitutes

Reducing sodium in your diet doesn't mean sacrificing taste. Explore these alternatives and substitutes to maintain flavor without excess salt:

Herb Blends: Create your own herb blends or use pre-made salt-free seasoning mixes to add depth and flavor to your dishes.

Vinegars: Balsamic, apple cider, and rice vinegar can add tanginess and complexity to your recipes without extra sodium.

Citrus Zest: Grate the zest of citrus fruits like lemon or orange to infuse dishes with natural, salt-free flavor.

Garlic and Onion: Utilize fresh or powdered garlic and onion to impart savory notes to your meals.

Mustard and Horseradish: These condiments can provide a flavorful punch without relying on salt.

Essential Kitchen Tools for Low Sodium Cooking

Equipping your kitchen with the right tools can make low sodium cooking more convenient and enjoyable:

Herb Grinder: Invest in a quality herb grinder to easily crush and blend fresh herbs, releasing their full flavor.

Citrus Juicer and Zester: Extract the maximum flavor from citrus fruits by using a juicer and zester to add zing to your dishes.

Non-Stick Cookware: Non-stick pans reduce the need for added fats and oils, allowing you to control your overall sodium and fat intake.

Steamer Basket: Steam vegetables to retain nutrients and enhance natural flavors without the need for added salt.

Quality Knives: A set of sharp knives makes it easier to work with fresh produce and meats, encouraging you to choose whole ingredients over processed ones.

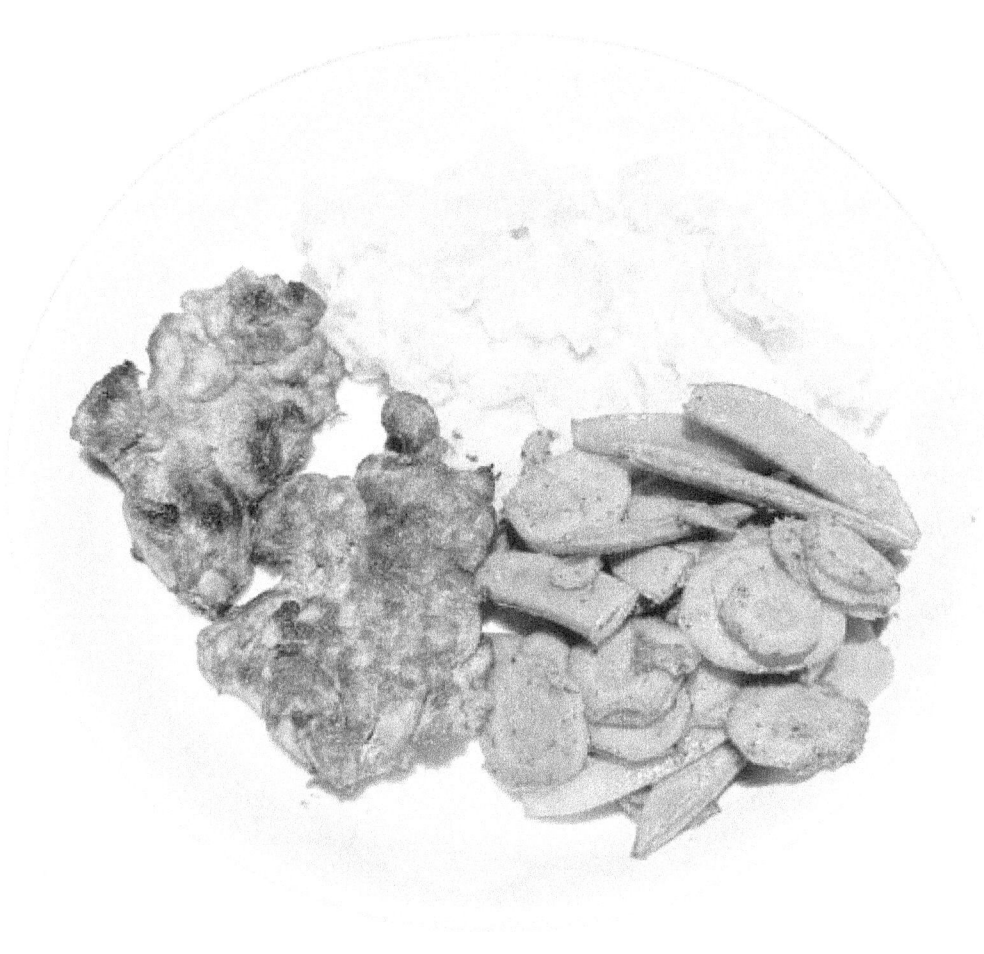

CHAPTER 3

BREAKFAST DELIGHTS

Avocado and Tomato Breakfast Sandwich

Cooking Time: 10 minutes

Serving: 1

Ingredients:

- ❖ 1 whole-grain English muffin
- ❖ 1/2 ripe avocado, mashed.
- ❖ 1 tomato, sliced.
- ❖ Salt-free seasoning

Instructions:

1. Toast the English muffin.
2. Spread mashed avocado on one half and layer with sliced tomatoes.
3. Sprinkle with salt-free seasoning.

Nutritional Information:

280 calories, 35g carbs, 7g protein, 14g fat, 8g fiber

This nutrient-packed breakfast provides healthy fats and a burst of freshness to kickstart your day.

Greek Yogurt Parfait with Berries

Cooking Time: 5 minutes

Serving: 1

Ingredients:

- ❖ 1 cup non-fat Greek yogurt
- ❖ 1/2 cup mixed berries (blueberries, strawberries)
- ❖ 1 tablespoon honey (optional)
- ❖ 1 tablespoon chopped nuts.

Instructions:

1. Layer Greek yogurt with berries in a glass.
2. Drizzle with honey and sprinkle with chopped nuts.

Nutritional Information:

220 calories, 30g carbs, 18g protein, 5g fat, 4g fiber

Packed with protein and antioxidants, this parfait is a tasty and energizing way to start your morning.

Spinach and Mushroom Omelet

Cooking Time: 15 minutes

Serving: 1

Ingredients:

- ❖ 2 eggs, beaten.
- ❖ Handful of spinach
- ❖ 1/2 cup sliced mushrooms.
- ❖ Salt-free seasoning

Instructions:

1. Sauté spinach and mushrooms until wilted.
2. Pour beaten eggs over the vegetables and cook until set.
3. Season with salt-free seasoning.

Nutritional Information:

180 calories, 8g carbs, 15g protein, 10g fat, 3g fiber

Packed with protein and veggies, this omelet is a low-calorie, nutrient-dense breakfast option.

Banana and Almond Butter Smoothie

Cooking Time: 5 minutes

Serving: 1

Ingredients:

- ❖ 1 ripe banana
- ❖ 1 tablespoon almond butter
- ❖ 1/2 cup almond milk (unsweetened)
- ❖ Ice cubes

Instructions:

1. Blend banana, almond butter, almond milk, and ice until smooth.

Nutritional Information:

280 calories, 35g carbs, 5g protein, 15g fat, 6g fiber

A delicious and creamy smoothie that provides a good balance of carbohydrates, healthy fats, and fiber.

Quinoa Breakfast Bowl

Cooking Time: 20 minutes

Serving: 1

Ingredients:

- ❖ 1/2 cup cooked quinoa
- ❖ 1/2 cup mixed berries
- ❖ 1 tablespoon chia seeds
- ❖ 1/4 cup low-fat milk

Instructions:

1. Combine cooked quinoa, mixed berries, chia seeds, and milk in a bowl.

Nutritional Information:

220 calories, 40g carbs, 7g protein, 4g fat, 8g fiber

A hearty and fiber-rich breakfast that keeps you full and energized throughout the morning.

Whole Grain Pancakes with Fruit Topping

Cooking Time: 15 minutes

Serving: 2

Ingredients:

- ❖ 1 cup whole wheat pancake mix
- ❖ 3/4 cup water
- ❖ 1 cup mixed fresh fruit (berries, sliced bananas)

Instructions:

1. Prepare pancake mix according to package instructions.
2. Cook pancakes and top with fresh fruit.

Nutritional Information:

250 calories, 50g carbs, 7g protein, 2g fat, 8g fiber

A wholesome and satisfying pancake breakfast with the goodness of whole grains and fresh fruit.

Sweet Potato and Egg Breakfast Hash

Cooking Time: 25 minutes

Serving: 1

Ingredients:

- ❖ 1 small, sweet potato, diced.
- ❖ 1/2 onion, diced.
- ❖ 1 bell pepper, chopped.
- ❖ 2 eggs

Instructions:

1. Sauté sweet potato, onion, and bell pepper until tender.
2. Create wells in the hash and crack eggs into each well.
3. Cover and cook until eggs are done.

Nutritional Information:

280 calories, 35g carbs, 12g protein, 10g fat, 6g fiber

A nutrient-dense, colorful breakfast that provides a balance of carbohydrates, protein, and vitamins.

Cottage Cheese and Pineapple Bowl

Cooking Time: 5 minutes

Serving: 1

Ingredients:

- ❖ 1/2 cup low-fat cottage cheese
- ❖ 1 cup fresh pineapple chunks
- ❖ 1 tablespoon shredded coconut

Instructions:

1. Combine cottage cheese, pineapple chunks, and shredded coconut in a bowl.

Nutritional Information:

220 calories, 30g carbs, 15g protein, 5g fat, 3g fiber

A quick and satisfying breakfast that provides protein, vitamin C, and a touch of tropical sweetness.

Egg White and Vegetable Wrap

Cooking Time: 10 minutes

Serving: 1

Ingredients:

- ❖ 2 egg whites, beaten.
- ❖ Handful of spinach
- ❖ 1/4 cup diced tomatoes.
- ❖ Whole grain wrap

Instructions:

1. Sauté spinach and tomatoes until wilted.
2. Pour beaten egg whites over the vegetables and cook until set.
3. Fill a whole grain wrap with the cooked egg whites and vegetables.

Nutritional Information:

220 calories, 30g carbs, 18g protein, 3g fat, 5g fiber

A low-calorie, high-protein wrap that's perfect for a quick and nutritious breakfast on the go.

Chia Seed Pudding with Mango

Cooking Time: 5 minutes (plus overnight soaking)

Serving: 1

Ingredients:

- ❖ 3 tablespoons chia seeds
- ❖ 1 cup unsweetened almond milk
- ❖ 1/2 teaspoon vanilla extract
- ❖ 1/2 cup diced mango.

Instructions:

1. Mix chia seeds, almond milk, and vanilla extract in a jar.
2. Refrigerate overnight.
3. Top with diced mango before serving.

Nutritional Information:

220 calories, 30g carbs, 5g protein, 10g fat, 10g fiber

A delicious and fiber-rich pudding that's not only satisfying but also a great source of omega-3 fatty acids.

CHAPTER 4

SATISFYING SOUPS AND STEWS

Vegetable and Lentil Soup

Cooking Time: 30 minutes

Serving: 4

Ingredients:

- ❖ 1 cup lentils, rinsed.
- ❖ 4 cups low-sodium vegetable broth
- ❖ 2 carrots, diced.
- ❖ 2 celery stalks, chopped.

Instructions:

1. Combine lentils, vegetable broth, carrots, and celery in a pot.
2. Simmer until lentils are tender.

Nutritional Information:

180 calories, 30g carbs, 12g protein, 1g fat, 8g fiber

Packed with plant-based protein and fiber, this soup is a nutritious and hearty option for a satisfying meal.

Chicken and Rice Soup

Cooking Time: 40 minutes

Serving: 6

Ingredients:

- ❖ 1 lb. boneless, skinless chicken breast
- ❖ 1 cup brown rice
- ❖ 4 cups low-sodium chicken broth
- ❖ 2 carrots, sliced.

Instructions:

1. Cook chicken in broth until done, shred, and return to the pot.
2. Add rice and carrots, simmer until rice is cooked.

Nutritional Information:

220 calories, 25g carbs, 25g protein, 3g fat, 3g fiber

A classic favorite, this low sodium chicken and rice soup offers comfort and a good balance of protein and carbohydrates.

Tomato Basil Quinoa Stew

Cooking Time: 35 minutes

Serving: 4

Ingredients:

- ❖ 1 cup quinoa, rinsed.
- ❖ 4 cups low-sodium vegetable broth
- ❖ 1 can (14 oz) diced tomatoes.
- ❖ Fresh basil leaves, chopped.

Instructions:

1. Combine quinoa, vegetable broth, and diced tomatoes in a pot.
2. Simmer until quinoa is cooked, stir in fresh basil before serving.

Nutritional Information:

250 calories, 45g carbs, 10g protein, 4g fat, 8g fiber

This stew combines the goodness of quinoa and tomatoes for a flavorful, nutrient-packed meal.

Mushroom and Barley Soup

Cooking Time: 45 minutes

Serving: 6

Ingredients:

- ❖ 1 cup pearl barley
- ❖ 5 cups low-sodium vegetable broth
- ❖ 1 lb. mushrooms, sliced.
- ❖ 1 onion, diced.

Instructions:

1. Cook barley in vegetable broth until almost tender.
2. Sauté mushrooms and onions, add to the pot and simmer until barley is fully cooked.

Nutritional Information:

180 calories, 40g carbs, 6g protein, 1g fat, 8g fiber

A hearty and earthy soup, the combination of mushrooms and barley provides a satisfying and wholesome experience.

Minestrone Soup

Cooking Time: 40 minutes

Serving: 8

Ingredients:

- ❖ 1 can (15 oz) kidney beans, drained.
- ❖ 1 cup whole wheat pasta, cooked.
- ❖ 4 cups low-sodium vegetable broth
- ❖ 1 zucchini, diced.

Instructions:

1. Combine kidney beans, cooked pasta, vegetable broth, and zucchini in a pot.
2. Simmer until the zucchini is tender.

Nutritional Information:

220 calories, 40g carbs, 10g protein, 2g fat, 6g fiber

This classic Italian soup is a colorful and nutritious medley of beans, pasta, and vegetables.

Lentil and Spinach Stew

Cooking Time: 30 minutes

Serving: 4

Ingredients:

- ❖ 1 cup green lentils, rinsed.
- ❖ 4 cups low-sodium vegetable broth
- ❖ 2 cups fresh spinach
- ❖ 1 onion, chopped.

Instructions:

1. Cook lentils and onion in vegetable broth until lentils are tender.
2. Stir in fresh spinach until wilted.

Nutritional Information:

190 calories, 30g carbs, 15g protein, 1g fat, 8g fiber

Packed with plant-based protein and iron, this stew is a nutritious and energizing option for a satisfying meal.

Sweet Potato and Black Bean Chili

Cooking Time: 35 minutes

Serving: 6

Ingredients:

- ❖ 2 sweet potatoes, diced.
- ❖ 2 cans (15 oz each) black beans, drained.
- ❖ 1 can (14 oz) diced tomatoes.
- ❖ 1 tablespoon chili powder

Instructions:

1. Combine sweet potatoes, black beans, diced tomatoes, and chili powder in a pot.
2. Simmer until sweet potatoes are tender.

Nutritional Information:

240 calories, 45g carbs, 12g protein, 1g fat, 10g fiber

A vibrant and flavorful chili that combines the sweetness of sweet potatoes with the protein-packed goodness of black beans.

Coconut Curry Lentil Soup

Cooking Time: 40 minutes

Serving: 4

Ingredients:

- ❖ 1 cup red lentils, rinsed.
- ❖ 1 can (14 oz) coconut milk
- ❖ 2 tablespoons curry powder
- ❖ 1 carrot, sliced.

Instructions:

1. Cook lentils and carrots in coconut milk with curry powder until lentils are tender.

Nutritional Information:

280 calories, 35g carbs, 15g protein, 10g fat, 8g fiber

A rich and aromatic soup that marries the creaminess of coconut milk with the warmth of curry spices.

Turkey and Vegetable Quinoa Soup

Cooking Time: 30 minutes

Serving: 6

Ingredients:

- ❖ 1 lb. ground turkey
- ❖ 1 cup quinoa, rinsed.
- ❖ 4 cups low-sodium chicken broth
- ❖ Mixed vegetables (carrots, peas, corn)

Instructions:

1. Brown turkey in a pot, add quinoa, mixed vegetables, and chicken broth.
2. Simmer until quinoa is cooked.

Nutritional Information:

240 calories, 25g carbs, 20g protein, 7g fat, 5g fiber

A protein-packed soup that combines the lean goodness of turkey with the nutritious benefits of quinoa and vegetables.

Butternut Squash and Apple Soup

Cooking Time: 45 minutes

Serving: 4

Ingredients:

- ❖ 1 butternut squash peeled and diced.
- ❖ 2 apples peeled and chopped.
- ❖ 4 cups low-sodium vegetable broth
- ❖ 1 teaspoon cinnamon

Instructions:

1. Cook butternut squash and apples in vegetable broth until tender.
2. Puree the mixture and add cinnamon before serving.

Nutritional Information:

180 calories, 40g carbs, 3g protein, 1g fat, 8g fiber

A delightful and vitamin-rich soup that blends the sweetness of apples with the savory notes of butternut squash.

CHAPTER 5

SALADS AND DRESSINGS

Mediterranean Chickpea Salad

Preparation Time: 15 minutes

Serving: 4

Ingredients:

- ❖ 2 cans (15 oz each) chickpeas, drained.
- ❖ 1 cucumber, diced.
- ❖ 1 cup cherry tomatoes, halved.
- ❖ Feta cheese, crumbled.

Instructions:

1. Combine chickpeas, cucumber, and cherry tomatoes in a bowl.
2. Top with crumbled feta cheese.

Nutritional Information:

220 calories, 35g carbs, 12g protein, 6g fat, 10g fiber

Bursting with flavors, this salad is rich in plant-based protein and fiber for a satisfying and nutritious meal.

Quinoa and Vegetable Salad

Preparation Time: 20 minutes

Serving: 4

Ingredients:

- ❖ 1 cup quinoa, cooked.
- ❖ 1 bell pepper, diced.
- ❖ 1 cup cucumber, sliced.
- ❖ 1/2 red onion finely chopped.

Instructions:

1. Mix cooked quinoa with diced bell pepper, sliced cucumber, and chopped red onion.

Nutritional Information:

240 calories, 40g carbs, 8g protein, 5g fat, 6g fiber

A nutrient-packed salad that combines the goodness of quinoa with a variety of colorful vegetables.

Grilled Chicken Caesar Salad

Preparation Time: 25 minutes

Serving: 2

Ingredients:

- ❖ 2 boneless, skinless chicken breasts
- ❖ Romaine lettuce, chopped.
- ❖ Cherry tomatoes, halved.
- ❖ Parmesan cheese, grated.

Instructions:

1. Grill chicken breasts until cooked, then slice.
2. Toss chopped Romaine lettuce with cherry tomatoes, top with grilled chicken, and sprinkle with Parmesan cheese.

Nutritional Information:

280 calories, 15g carbs, 35g protein, 8g fat, 5g fiber

Motivation: A classic favorite made healthier; this grilled chicken Caesar salad is a protein-packed delight.

Avocado and Black Bean Salad

Preparation Time: 15 minutes

Serving: 4

Ingredients:

- ❖ 2 avocados, diced.
- ❖ 1 can (15 oz) black beans drained and rinsed.
- ❖ 1 cup corn kernels (fresh or frozen)
- ❖ Fresh cilantro, chopped.

Instructions:

1. Combine diced avocados, black beans, corn, and chopped cilantro in a bowl.

Nutritional Information:

230 calories, 30g carbs, 8g protein, 11g fat, 9g fiber

Packed with heart-healthy fats and fiber, this salad is a tasty and satisfying choice.

Spinach and Strawberry Salad

Preparation Time: 10 minutes

Serving: 4

Ingredients:

- ❖ Fresh spinach leaves
- ❖ Strawberries, sliced.
- ❖ Goat cheese, crumbled.
- ❖ Balsamic vinaigrette dressing

Instructions:

1. Toss fresh spinach with sliced strawberries, crumbled goat cheese, and drizzle with balsamic vinaigrette.

Nutritional Information:

180 calories, 20g carbs, 7g protein, 9g fat, 5g fiber

A delightful combination of sweet and savory, this salad is rich in antioxidants and vitamins.

Tuna and White Bean Salad

Preparation Time: 15 minutes

Serving: 2

Ingredients:

- ❖ 2 cans (5 oz each) tuna, drained.
- ❖ 1 can (15 oz) white beans drained and rinsed.
- ❖ Red onion finely chopped.
- ❖ Cherry tomatoes, halved.

Instructions:

1. Mix tuna, white beans, chopped red onion, and cherry tomatoes in a bowl.

Nutritional Information:

250 calories, 25g carbs, 30g protein, 5g fat, 8g fiber

A protein-packed salad that combines the lean goodness of tuna with the fiber-rich white beans.

Cucumber and Dill Greek Salad

Preparation Time: 15 minutes

Serving: 4

Ingredients:

- ❖ English cucumber, sliced.
- ❖ Kalamata olives, pitted.
- ❖ Feta cheese, crumbled.
- ❖ Fresh dill, chopped.

Instructions:

1. Combine sliced cucumber, Kalamata olives, crumbled feta cheese, and chopped fresh dill in a bowl.

Nutritional Information:

200 calories, 15g carbs, 8g protein, 14g fat, 5g fiber

Transport your taste buds to the Mediterranean with this refreshing and flavorful Greek salad.

Roasted Vegetable Quinoa Salad

Preparation Time: 30 minutes

Serving: 4

Ingredients:

- ❖ 1 cup quinoa, cooked.
- ❖ Assorted vegetables (bell peppers, zucchini, cherry tomatoes), roasted.
- ❖ Balsamic vinaigrette dressing
- ❖ Fresh basil, chopped.

Instructions:

1. Mix cooked quinoa with roasted vegetables, drizzle with balsamic vinaigrette, and sprinkle with fresh basil.

Nutritional Information:

230 calories, 35g carbs, 6g protein, 8g fat, 5g fiber

This colorful and nutrient-packed salad is a celebration of roasted vegetables and wholesome quinoa.

Asian-Inspired Edamame Salad

Preparation Time: 20 minutes

Serving: 4

Ingredients:

- ❖ Edamame beans, cooked.
- ❖ Red cabbage thinly sliced.
- ❖ Carrots, shredded.
- ❖ Sesame ginger dressing

Instructions:

1. Combine cooked edamame beans, sliced red cabbage, and shredded carrots in a bowl.
2. Drizzle with sesame ginger dressing.

Nutritional Information:

190 calories, 20g carbs, 12g protein, 8g fat, 6g fiber

Packed with plant-based protein, this Asian-inspired salad is both satisfying and full of vibrant flavors.

Caprese Salad with Pesto Dressing

Preparation Time: 15 minutes

Serving: 2

Ingredients:

- ❖ Fresh mozzarella, sliced.
- ❖ Tomatoes, sliced.
- ❖ Fresh basil leaves
- ❖ Pesto dressing

Instructions:

1. Arrange sliced mozzarella, tomatoes, and fresh basil on a plate.
2. Drizzle with pesto dressing.

Nutritional Information:

250 calories, 6g carbs, 12g protein, 20g fat, 2g fiber

A classic Caprese salad elevated with the rich flavors of fresh mozzarella and aromatic pesto dressing.

CHAPTER 6

WHOLESOME MAIN COURSES

Baked Lemon Herb Chicken

Cooking Time: 40 minutes

Serving: 4

Ingredients:

- ❖ 4 boneless, skinless chicken breasts
- ❖ 1 lemon juiced and zested.
- ❖ Fresh herbs (rosemary, thyme)
- ❖ Olive oil

Instructions:

1. Marinate chicken in lemon juice, zest, herbs, and olive oil.
2. Bake until chicken is cooked through.

Nutritional Information:

240 calories, 2g carbs, 30g protein, 12g fat, 1g fiber

A simple yet flavorful dish, this baked chicken is a protein powerhouse with a burst of citrusy freshness.

Salmon and Quinoa Bowl

Cooking Time: 25 minutes

Serving: 2

Ingredients:

- ❖ 2 salmon fillets
- ❖ 1 cup quinoa, cooked.
- ❖ Steamed broccoli.
- ❖ Lemon wedges

Instructions:

1. Grill or bake salmon fillets.
2. Serve over a bed of cooked quinoa with steamed broccoli, garnish with lemon wedges.

Nutritional Information:

320 calories, 30g carbs, 30g protein, 10g fat, 5g fiber

A nutrient-rich bowl that combines omega-3 rich salmon with protein-packed quinoa for a satisfying and wholesome meal.

Stir-Fried Tofu and Vegetable Quinoa

Cooking Time: 30 minutes

Serving: 4

Ingredients:

- ❖ 1 block firm tofu, cubed.
- ❖ Mixed vegetables (bell peppers, broccoli, carrots)
- ❖ 1 cup quinoa, cooked.
- ❖ Low-sodium soy sauce

Instructions:

- ❖ Sauté tofu and mixed vegetables in a pan, stir in cooked quinoa, and add soy sauce to taste.

Nutritional Information:

280 calories, 35g carbs, 15g protein, 10g fat, 6g fiber

A plant-based delight, this stir-fry offers a balance of protein, fiber, and vibrant vegetables.

Baked Cod with Herbed Quinoa

Cooking Time: 25 minutes

Serving: 4

Ingredients:

- ❖ 4 cod fillets
- ❖ 1 cup quinoa, cooked.
- ❖ Fresh herbs (parsley, dill)
- ❖ Lemon slices

Instructions:

1. Place cod fillets on a baking sheet, season with herbs, and bake.
2. Serve over a bed of herbed quinoa, garnish with lemon slices.

Nutritional Information:

260 calories, 20g carbs, 30g protein, 8g fat, 3g fiber

A light and flavorful dish, this baked cod with herbed quinoa is a perfect balance of protein and wholesome grains.

Vegetarian Chickpea Curry

Cooking Time: 30 minutes

Serving: 4

Ingredients:

- ❖ 2 cans (15 oz each) chickpeas, drained.
- ❖ 1 can (14 oz) diced tomatoes.
- ❖ Onion, diced.
- ❖ Curry spices (cumin, coriander, turmeric)

Instructions:

1. Sauté diced onion, add chickpeas, diced tomatoes, and curry spices.
2. Simmer until flavors meld.

Nutritional Information:

280 calories, 45g carbs, 14g protein, 5g fat, 12g fiber

Packed with plant-based protein and fiber, this chickpea curry is a flavorful and satisfying meatless option.

Turkey and Vegetable Skewers

Cooking Time: 20 minutes

Serving: 4

Ingredients:

- ❖ 1 lb. ground turkey
- ❖ Bell peppers, cherry tomatoes, zucchini (cut into chunks)
- ❖ Olive oil
- ❖ Italian seasoning

Instructions:

1. Mix ground turkey with Italian seasoning, shape into skewers, and thread with vegetables.
2. Grill or bake until turkey is cooked through.

Nutritional Information:

240 calories, 15g carbs, 30g protein, 8g fat, 3g fiber

These flavorful turkey and vegetable skewers are a lean and protein-packed option for a satisfying meal.

Shrimp and Broccoli Stir-Fry

Cooking Time: 20 minutes

Serving: 3

Ingredients:

- ❖ 1 lb. shrimp peeled and deveined.
- ❖ Broccoli florets
- ❖ Low-sodium soy sauce
- ❖ Garlic, minced.

Instructions:

1. Sauté shrimp and broccoli in a pan with minced garlic, add soy sauce to taste.

Nutritional Information:

200 calories, 10g carbs, 25g protein, 7g fat, 4g fiber

Quick and easy, this shrimp and broccoli stir-fry is a delicious way to incorporate lean protein and vegetables.

Lemon Garlic Roast Chicken

Cooking Time: 1 hour

Serving: 6

Ingredients:

- ❖ 1 whole chicken
- ❖ 2 lemons, sliced.
- ❖ Garlic cloves, minced.
- ❖ Olive oil

Instructions:

1. Rub the chicken with minced garlic, olive oil, and lemon slices.
2. Roast until the chicken reaches an internal temperature of 165°F.

Nutritional Information:

280 calories, 2g carbs, 35g protein, 14g fat, 0g fiber

This lemon garlic roast chicken is not only simple to prepare but also a flavorful and comforting main course.

Spaghetti Squash with Turkey Bolognese

Cooking Time: 45 minutes

Serving: 4

Ingredients:

- ❖ 1 medium spaghetti squash
- ❖ 1 lb. ground turkey
- ❖ Low-sodium marinara sauce
- ❖ Fresh basil, chopped.

Instructions:

1. Roast spaghetti squash, sauté ground turkey, and mix with marinara sauce.
2. Serve turkey Bolognese over the roasted spaghetti squash, garnish with fresh basil.

Nutritional Information:

300 calories, 35g carbs, 25g protein, 10g fat, 8g fiber

A healthier twist on a classic, this spaghetti squash with turkey Bolognese is a low-carb and protein-rich alternative.

Vegetable and Tofu Stir-Fry

Cooking Time: 25 minutes

Serving: 3

Ingredients:

- ❖ 1 block firm tofu, cubed.
- ❖ Mixed vegetables (bell peppers, snap peas, carrots)
- ❖ Low-sodium stir-fry sauce
- ❖ Brown rice, cooked.

Instructions:

1. Sauté tofu and mixed vegetables in a pan, add stir-fry sauce, and serve over cooked brown rice.

Nutritional Information:

250 calories, 35g carbs, 15g protein, 8g fat, 6g fiber

A colorful and wholesome stir-fry that brings together tofu, crisp vegetables, and nutrient-rich brown rice.

Baked Sweet Potato and Black Bean Enchiladas

Cooking Time: 45 minutes

Serving: 4

Ingredients:

- ❖ 2 sweet potatoes, mashed.
- ❖ 1 can (15 oz) black beans drained and mashed.
- ❖ Whole wheat tortillas
- ❖ Enchilada sauce (low sodium)

Instructions:

1. Fill tortillas with mashed sweet potatoes and black beans, roll, and place in a baking dish.
2. Pour enchilada sauce over the top and bake until bubbly.

Nutritional Information:

280 calories, 50g carbs, 10g protein, 5g fat, 12g fiber

These enchiladas are a tasty, plant-based alternative that's high in fiber and flavor.

Mushroom and Spinach Quiche with Oat Crust

Cooking Time: 40 minutes

Serving: 6

Ingredients:

- ❖ Oat crust (oats, olive oil)
- ❖ 1 cup mushrooms, sliced.
- ❖ 2 cups fresh spinach
- ❖ 6 eggs, beaten.

Instructions:

1. Press oat crust into a pie dish, sauté mushrooms and spinach, place in the crust, and pour beaten eggs over.
2. Bake until eggs are set.

Nutritional Information:

220 calories, 15g carbs, 15g protein, 12g fat, 4g fiber

A nutritious quiche that swaps traditional crust for a wholesome oat alternative.

Teriyaki Salmon with Brown Rice

Cooking Time: 25 minutes

Serving: 4

Ingredients:

- ❖ 4 salmon fillets
- ❖ Low-sodium teriyaki sauce
- ❖ Brown rice, cooked.
- ❖ Steamed broccoli.

Instructions:

1. Marinate salmon in teriyaki sauce, grill or bake until cooked.
2. Serve over brown rice with steamed broccoli.

Nutritional Information:

300 calories, 30g carbs, 25g protein, 10g fat, 4g fiber

A flavorful and protein-packed dish that combines the goodness of salmon with whole grains.

Vegetarian Stuffed Bell Peppers

Cooking Time: 50 minutes

Serving: 6

Ingredients:

- ❖ Bell peppers, halved.
- ❖ Quinoa, cooked.
- ❖ Black beans drained and rinsed.
- ❖ Diced tomatoes, onion, and corn.

Instructions:

1. Mix quinoa, black beans, diced tomatoes, onion, and corn, stuff into halved bell peppers, and bake.

Nutritional Information:

260 calories, 40g carbs, 10g protein, 5g fat, 8g fiber

These stuffed peppers offer a colorful and nutritious way to enjoy a variety of veggies and plant-based protein.

Lemon Garlic Shrimp and Asparagus Pasta

Cooking Time: 30 minutes

Serving: 4

Ingredients:

- ❖ 1 lb. shrimp peeled and deveined.
- ❖ Whole wheat pasta
- ❖ Asparagus trimmed and sliced.
- ❖ Lemon, garlic, olive oil

Instructions:

1. Sauté shrimp and asparagus in a pan with minced garlic and olive oil.
2. Toss with cooked whole wheat pasta and lemon juice.

Nutritional Information:

320 calories, 40g carbs, 25g protein, 8g fat, 6g fiber

A light and zesty pasta dish that features the freshness of shrimp, asparagus, and citrus.

Eggplant and Chickpea Tagine

Cooking Time: 40 minutes

Serving: 4

Ingredients:

- ❖ Eggplant, diced.
- ❖ 1 can (15 oz) chickpeas, drained.
- ❖ Diced tomatoes.
- ❖ Moroccan spices (cumin, coriander, cinnamon)

Instructions:

1. Sauté diced eggplant, add chickpeas, diced tomatoes, and spices, simmer until flavors meld.

Nutritional Information:

230 calories, 35g carbs, 10g protein, 8g fat, 10g fiber

Transport your taste buds with this aromatic and fiber-rich eggplant and chickpea tagine.

Turkey and Vegetable Meatball Subs

Cooking Time: 30 minutes

Serving: 4

Ingredients:

- ❖ 1 lb. ground turkey
- ❖ Zucchini, carrots, and onion (grated)
- ❖ Whole wheat sub rolls
- ❖ Marinara sauce (low sodium)

Instructions:

1. Mix ground turkey with grated vegetables, form into meatballs, bake until cooked.
2. Serve meatballs in whole wheat sub rolls with marinara sauce.

Nutritional Information:

280 calories, 30g carbs, 25g protein, 8g fat, 6g fiber

A healthier take on a classic, these turkey and vegetable meatball subs are a tasty and nutritious option.

Chickpea and Spinach Coconut Curry

Cooking Time: 35 minutes

Serving: 4

Ingredients:

- ❖ 2 cans (15 oz each) chickpeas, drained.
- ❖ Fresh spinach
- ❖ Coconut milk
- ❖ Curry spices (turmeric, cumin, coriander)

Instructions:

1. Simmer chickpeas, fresh spinach, coconut milk, and curry spices until heated through.

Nutritional Information:

290 calories, 40g carbs, 12g protein, 10g fat, 8g fiber

This chickpea and spinach coconut curry offers a creamy and flavorful plant-based meal.

Cauliflower and Lentil Tacos

Cooking Time: 30 minutes

Serving: 6

Ingredients:

- ❖ Cauliflower florets, roasted.
- ❖ Lentils, cooked.
- ❖ Whole wheat tortillas
- ❖ Taco toppings (salsa, avocado, cilantro)

Instructions:

1. Fill tortillas with roasted cauliflower, cooked lentils, and desired toppings.

Nutritional Information:

240 calories, 35g carbs, 10g protein, 8g fat, 8g fiber

These cauliflower and lentil tacos are a delicious and fiber-packed twist on traditional tacos.

Sesame Ginger Chicken Stir-Fry

Cooking Time: 25 minutes

Serving: 4

Ingredients:

- ❖ 1 lb chicken breast, sliced.
- ❖ Mixed vegetables (bell peppers, snow peas, carrots)
- ❖ Low-sodium sesame ginger stir-fry sauce
- ❖ Brown rice, cooked.

Instructions:

1. Stir-fry chicken and mixed vegetables in a pan, add stir-fry sauce, and serve over cooked brown rice.

Nutritional Information:

290 calories, 35g carbs, 25g protein, 6g fat, 4g fiber

A quick and flavorful stir-fry that brings together lean protein, crisp vegetables, and whole grains.

CHAPTER 7

SNACKS AND APPETIZERS

Guacamole with Veggie Sticks

Preparation Time: 15 minutes

Serving: 4

Ingredients:

- ❖ 3 ripe avocados, mashed.
- ❖ Tomatoes, onion, cilantro (diced)
- ❖ Lime juice
- ❖ Carrot and cucumber sticks

Instructions:

1. Mix mashed avocados with diced tomatoes, onion, cilantro, and lime juice.
2. Serve with carrot and cucumber sticks.

Nutritional Information:

180 calories, 15g carbs, 3g protein, 14g fat, 7g fiber

Guacamole is a nutrient-packed dip that pairs perfectly with fresh and crunchy veggies for a satisfying snack.

Baked Zucchini Chips

Preparation Time: 20 minutes

Serving: 2

Ingredients:

- ❖ Zucchini thinly sliced.
- ❖ Olive oil
- ❖ Parmesan cheese (optional)
- ❖ Paprika and garlic powder

Instructions:

1. Toss zucchini slices with olive oil, paprika, and garlic powder.
2. Bake until crispy and sprinkle with Parmesan cheese if desired.

Nutritional Information:

120 calories, 10g carbs, 2g protein, 8g fat, 3g fiber

These baked zucchini chips are a flavorful alternative to traditional chips, offering a satisfying crunch.

Hummus and Veggie Platter

Preparation Time: 15 minutes

Serving: 4

Ingredients:

- ❖ Hummus (store-bought or homemade)
- ❖ Cherry tomatoes, cucumber slices, bell pepper strips
- ❖ Whole grain pita wedges

Instructions:

1. Arrange hummus, cherry tomatoes, cucumber slices, and bell pepper strips on a platter.
2. Serve with whole grain pita wedges.

Nutritional Information:

180 calories, 25g carbs, 6g protein, 7g fat, 6g fiber

A hummus and veggie platter is a colorful and nutrient-rich snack that provides a satisfying combination of flavors.

Apple and Almond Butter Slices

Preparation Time: 5 minutes

Serving: 2

Ingredients:

- ❖ Apples thinly sliced.
- ❖ Almond butter
- ❖ Chia seeds (optional)
- ❖ Cinnamon

Instructions:

1. Spread almond butter on apple slices, sprinkle with chia seeds and cinnamon.

Nutritional Information:

160 calories, 18g carbs, 3g protein, 9g fat, 5g fiber

A simple and satisfying snack, apple and almond butter slices offer a combination of sweetness and crunch.

Caprese Skewers

Preparation Time: 15 minutes

Serving: 4

Ingredients:

- ❖ Cherry tomatoes
- ❖ Fresh mozzarella balls
- ❖ Basil leaves
- ❖ Balsamic glaze

Instructions:

1. Thread cherry tomatoes, fresh mozzarella balls, and basil leaves onto skewers.
2. Drizzle with balsamic glaze before serving.

Nutritional Information:

160 calories, 5g carbs, 8g protein, 12g fat, 1g fiber

These Caprese skewers are a delightful and elegant snack, showcasing the classic combination of tomatoes, mozzarella, and basil.

Trail Mix with Nuts and Dried Fruits

Preparation Time: 5 minutes

Serving: 6

Ingredients:

- ❖ Mixed nuts (almonds, walnuts, cashews)
- ❖ Dried fruits (apricots, cranberries)
- ❖ Dark chocolate chunks
- ❖ Pumpkin seeds

Instructions:

1. Mix nuts, dried fruits, dark chocolate chunks, and pumpkin seeds in a bowl.

Nutritional Information:

200 calories, 20g carbs, 6g protein, 12g fat, 4g fiber

Trail mix is a versatile and portable snack that provides a mix of energy-boosting nuts and sweet dried fruits.

Cucumber Sushi Rolls

Preparation Time: 20 minutes

Serving: 4

Ingredients:

- ❖ Cucumbers thinly sliced.
- ❖ Avocado, julienned.
- ❖ Carrots, julienned.
- ❖ Smoked salmon (optional)

Instructions:

1. Lay cucumber slices flat, add julienned avocado, carrots, and smoked salmon (if using).
2. Roll up and secure with toothpicks.

Nutritional Information:

140 calories, 10g carbs, 3g protein, 8g fat, 3g fiber

Cucumber sushi rolls are a refreshing and low-calorie alternative to traditional sushi, perfect for a light snack.

Quinoa Salad Cups

Preparation Time: 25 minutes

Serving: 8

Ingredients:

- ❖ Mini phyllo cups
- ❖ Quinoa, cooked.
- ❖ Cherry tomatoes, cucumber, feta cheese
- ❖ Balsamic glaze

Instructions:

1. Fill mini phyllo cups with cooked quinoa, diced cherry tomatoes, cucumber, and crumbled feta.
2. Drizzle with balsamic glaze.

Nutritional Information:

120 calories, 15g carbs, 4g protein, 6g fat, 2g fiber

Quinoa salad cups are a delightful and bite-sized way to enjoy a nutritious mix of whole grains and fresh vegetables.

Stuffed Bell Pepper Bites

Preparation Time: 30 minutes

Serving: 6

Ingredients:

- ❖ Mini bell peppers, halved.
- ❖ Hummus
- ❖ Cherry tomatoes, diced.
- ❖ Fresh parsley, chopped.

Instructions:

1. Fill mini bell pepper halves with hummus, top with diced cherry tomatoes and chopped fresh parsley.

Nutritional Information:

100 calories, 12g carbs, 3g protein, 5g fat, 3g fiber

Stuffed bell pepper bites are a colorful and flavorful snack that combines the freshness of vegetables with the creaminess of hummus.

Mango Salsa with Whole Grain Pita Chips

Preparation Time: 15 minutes

Serving: 4

Ingredients:

- ❖ 2 ripe mangoes, diced.
- ❖ Red onion finely chopped.
- ❖ Fresh cilantro, chopped.
- ❖ Jalapeño seeded and minced.
- ❖ Lime juice
- ❖ Whole grain pita bread, cut into wedges.

Instructions:

1. In a bowl, combine diced mangoes, chopped red onion, cilantro, minced jalapeño, and lime juice. Mix well.
2. Toast whole grain pita wedges until crisp.
3. Serve the mango salsa with the whole grain pita chips.

Nutritional Information:

150 calories, 35g carbs, 2g protein, 1g fat, 5g fiber

This vibrant mango salsa with whole grain pita chips is a refreshing and nutritious snack that combines the sweetness of mangoes with a hint of spice for a delightful flavor experience.

CHAPTER 8

21 DAY MEAL PLAN

Day 1:

- ❖ Breakfast: Veggie Omelet with Whole Grain Toast
- ❖ Lunch: Baked Sweet Potato and Black Bean Enchiladas
- ❖ Dinner: Lemon Garlic Shrimp and Asparagus Pasta
- ❖ Snack: Guacamole with Veggie Sticks

Day 2:

- ❖ Breakfast: Greek Yogurt Parfait with Mixed Berries and Granola
- ❖ Lunch: Chickpea and Spinach Coconut Curry
- ❖ Dinner: Eggplant and Chickpea Tagine
- ❖ Snack: Berry Beet Boost Juice

Day 3:

- ❖ Breakfast: Spinach and Feta Omelet with Whole Grain Toast
- ❖ Lunch: Caprese Skewers
- ❖ Dinner: Teriyaki Salmon with Brown Rice
- ❖ Snack: Baked Zucchini Chips

Day 4:

- ❖ Breakfast: Whole Wheat Banana Nut Muffins
- ❖ Lunch: Quinoa Salad Cups
- ❖ Dinner: Mushroom and Spinach Quiche with Oat Crust
- ❖ Snack: Pomegranate Passion Juice

Day 5:

- ❖ Breakfast: Blueberry Almond Smoothie Bowl
- ❖ Lunch: Turkey and Vegetable Meatball Subs
- ❖ Dinner: Sesame Ginger Chicken Stir-Fry
- ❖ Snack: Hummus and Veggie Platter

Day 6:

- ❖ Breakfast: Avocado Toast with Poached Egg
- ❖ Lunch: Quinoa Salad Cups
- ❖ Dinner: Chickpea and Spinach Coconut Curry
- ❖ Snack: Greek Yogurt and Berry Parfait

Day 7:

- ❖ Breakfast: Whole Wheat Pancakes with Fresh Fruit Toppings
- ❖ Lunch: Caprese Skewers
- ❖ Dinner: Lemon Garlic Shrimp and Asparagus Pasta
- ❖ Snack: Baked Zucchini Chips

Day 8:

- ❖ Breakfast: Blueberry Almond Smoothie Bowl
- ❖ Lunch: Teriyaki Salmon with Brown Rice
- ❖ Dinner: Stuffed Bell Pepper Bites
- ❖ Snack: Mango Salsa with Whole Grain Pita Chips

Day 9:

- ❖ Breakfast: Veggie Omelet with Whole Grain Toast
- ❖ Lunch: Baked Sweet Potato and Black Bean Enchiladas
- ❖ Dinner: Eggplant and Chickpea Tagine
- ❖ Snack: Guacamole with Veggie Sticks

Day 10:

- ❖ Breakfast: Greek Yogurt Parfait with Mixed Berries and Granola
- ❖ Lunch: Chickpea and Spinach Coconut Curry
- ❖ Dinner: Teriyaki Salmon with Brown Rice
- ❖ Snack: Berry Beet Boost Juice

Day 11:

- ❖ Breakfast: Spinach and Feta Omelet with Whole Grain Toast
- ❖ Lunch: Caprese Skewers
- ❖ Dinner: Mushroom and Spinach Quiche with Oat Crust
- ❖ Snack: Pomegranate Passion Juice

Day 12:

- ❖ Breakfast: Whole Wheat Banana Nut Muffins
- ❖ Lunch: Quinoa Salad Cups
- ❖ Dinner: Sesame Ginger Chicken Stir-Fry
- ❖ Snack: Hummus and Veggie Platter

Day 13:

- ❖ Breakfast: Avocado Toast with Poached Egg
- ❖ Lunch: Teriyaki Salmon with Brown Rice
- ❖ Dinner: Lemon Garlic Shrimp and Asparagus Pasta
- ❖ Snack: Mango Salsa with Whole Grain Pita Chips

Day 14:

- ❖ Breakfast: Blueberry Almond Smoothie Bowl
- ❖ Lunch: Quinoa Salad Cups
- ❖ Dinner: Stuffed Bell Pepper Bites
- ❖ Snack: Greek Yogurt and Berry Parfait

Day 15:

- ❖ Breakfast: Whole Wheat Pancakes with Fresh Fruit Toppings
- ❖ Lunch: Caprese Skewers
- ❖ Dinner: Chickpea and Spinach Coconut Curry
- ❖ Snack: Baked Zucchini Chips

Day 16:

- ❖ Breakfast: Blueberry Almond Smoothie Bowl
- ❖ Lunch: Turkey and Vegetable Meatball Subs
- ❖ Dinner: Mushroom and Spinach Quiche with Oat Crust
- ❖ Snack: Hummus and Veggie Platter

Day 17:

- ❖ Breakfast: Avocado Toast with Poached Egg
- ❖ Lunch: Baked Sweet Potato and Black Bean Enchiladas
- ❖ Dinner: Stuffed Bell Pepper Bites
- ❖ Snack: Mango Salsa with Whole Grain Pita Chips

Day 18:

- ❖ Breakfast: Greek Yogurt Parfait with Mixed Berries and Granola
- ❖ Lunch: Quinoa Salad Cups
- ❖ Dinner: Sesame Ginger Chicken Stir-Fry
- ❖ Snack: Berry Beet Boost Juice

Day 19:

- ❖ Breakfast: Whole Wheat Banana Nut Muffins
- ❖ Lunch: Caprese Skewers
- ❖ Dinner: Lemon Garlic Shrimp and Asparagus Pasta
- ❖ Snack: Baked Zucchini Chips

Day 20:

- ❖ Breakfast: Blueberry Almond Smoothie Bowl
- ❖ Lunch: Teriyaki Salmon with Brown Rice
- ❖ Dinner: Eggplant and Chickpea Tagine
- ❖ Snack: Hummus and Veggie Platter

Day 21:

- ❖ Breakfast: Avocado Toast with Poached Egg
- ❖ Lunch: Baked Sweet Potato and Black Bean Enchiladas
- ❖ Dinner: Stuffed Bell Pepper Bites
- ❖ Snack: Mango Salsa with Whole Grain Pita Chips

CONCLUSION

As we reach the end of this culinary voyage, I want to extend my heartfelt gratitude for joining me on this journey to savoring life through the lens of heart-healthy, low sodium delights. Together, we've explored the artistry of flavors, the simplicity of nourishing our bodies, and the profound joy that comes from embracing a lifestyle that champions well-being.

As Nutrionist Lorene Peachey, my hope is that this cookbook not only becomes a staple in your kitchen but a cherished companion on your path to a healthier, more vibrant you. The recipes within these pages are not mere instructions; they are invitations to create moments – moments of joy, discovery, and connection.

I would be remiss not to mention the importance of your feedback. Your experiences, your stories, and your insights are the heartbeat of this cookbook. As you embark on your culinary adventures, I encourage you to share your thoughts, your triumphs, and even the challenges you may encounter. Let your voice become a part of this narrative.

Did you discover a new favorite recipe that lit up your taste buds? Were there moments of revelation as you embraced the variety and simplicity of these low sodium delights? Your feedback is not just valuable; it's the soul of this culinary journey.

Remember, this cookbook is a living, breathing entity, and it thrives on the shared experiences of a community passionate about health and flavor. Your insights will not only shape the future editions but will also inspire others who follow in your culinary footsteps.

So, my dear friend, as you embark on your next kitchen escapade, let the spirit of exploration guide you. Cherish the flavors, celebrate the victories, and even find joy in the occasional mishap – for in those moments, culinary magic is often born.

As you close the pages of "Low Sodium Cookbook for Beginners," may you carry with you not just a cookbook but a newfound appreciation for the art of cooking and the profound impact it can have on our well-being.

Thank you for allowing me, Nutrionist Lorene Peachey, to be a part of your culinary expedition. Here's to a life filled with vibrant health, culinary exploration, and the endless joy of savoring each moment.

Wishing you countless delightful moments in your kitchen and a future filled with the savory richness of life.

BONUS CHAPTER:

JUICING FOR HEART HEALTHY

Citrus Bliss

Preparation Time: 10 minutes

Serving: 2

Ingredients:

- ❖ 2 oranges, peeled.
- ❖ 1 grapefruit, peeled.
- ❖ 1 lemon, peeled.

Instructions:

1. Juice oranges, grapefruit, and lemon.
2. Stir well and serve over ice.

Nutritional Information:

120 calories, 30g carbs, 2g protein, 0g fat, 5g fiber

Citrus fruits are rich in vitamin C and antioxidants, promoting heart health and a refreshing taste.

Berry Beet Boost

Preparation Time: 15 minutes

Serving: 2

Ingredients:

- ❖ 1 cup mixed berries (blueberries, strawberries)
- ❖ 1 small beet, peeled.
- ❖ 1 apple, cored.

Instructions:

1. Juice berries, beet, and apple.
2. Pour into glasses and enjoy.

Nutritional Information:

140 calories, 35g carbs, 2g protein, 0g fat, 8g fiber

Berries and beets provide a colorful blend of antioxidants and nutrients that support heart health.

Green Heart Elixir

Preparation Time: 12 minutes

Serving: 2

Ingredients:

- ❖ Handful of kale
- ❖ 1 cucumber
- ❖ 2 green apples, cored.

Instructions:

1. Juice kale, cucumber, and green apples.
2. Serve chilled with a slice of cucumber for garnish.

Nutritional Information:

100 calories, 25g carbs, 2g protein, 0g fat, 5g fiber

The chlorophyll in kale and the hydration from cucumber contribute to heart health and overall well-being.

Pomegranate Passion

Preparation Time: 10 minutes

Serving: 2

Ingredients:

- ❖ 1 cup pomegranate seeds
- ❖ 2 oranges, peeled.
- ❖ 1-inch ginger, peeled

Instructions:

1. Juice pomegranate seeds, oranges, and ginger.
2. Stir gently and pour into glasses.

Nutritional Information:

130 calories, 30g carbs, 2g protein, 1g fat, 6g fiber

Pomegranates contain powerful antioxidants that may contribute to heart health and overall cardiovascular wellness.

Turmeric Citrus Splash

Preparation Time: 12 minutes

Serving: 2

Ingredients:

- ❖ 2 oranges, peeled.
- ❖ 1 grapefruit, peeled.
- ❖ 1-inch turmeric root, peeled

Instructions:

1. Juice oranges, grapefruit, and turmeric.
2. Pour over ice and stir gently.

Nutritional Information:

110 calories, 28g carbs, 2g protein, 0.5g fat, 4g fiber

Turmeric's anti-inflammatory properties combined with citrus make this juice a heart-healthy powerhouse.

Carrot Ginger Zing

Preparation Time: 10 minutes

Serving: 2

Ingredients:

- ❖ 4 large carrots, peeled.
- ❖ 1 apple, cored.
- ❖ 1-inch ginger, peeled

Instructions:

1. Juice carrots, apple, and ginger.
2. Pour into glasses and enjoy the zing.

Nutritional Information:

120 calories, 30g carbs, 2g protein, 0g fat, 6g fiber

Carrots and ginger provide a vibrant mix of flavors and heart-boosting nutrients.

Heart Beet Fusion

Preparation Time: 15 minutes

Serving: 2

Ingredients:

- ❖ 2 beets, peeled.
- ❖ 1 cup pineapple chunks
- ❖ 1 orange, peeled.

Instructions:

1. Juice beets, pineapple, and orange.
2. Chill and serve over ice.

Nutritional Information:

140 calories, 35g carbs, 2g protein, 0.5g fat, 7g fiber

Beets, known for their nitrates, may contribute to lower blood pressure and heart health.

Minty Melon Refresher

Preparation Time: 12 minutes

Serving: 2

Ingredients:

- ❖ 2 cups watermelon, cubed.
- ❖ 1 cup honeydew melon, cubed.
- ❖ Fresh mint leaves

Instructions:

1. Juice watermelon and honeydew melon.
2. Garnish with fresh mint leaves.

Nutritional Information:

90 calories, 22g carbs, 1g protein, 0.5g fat, 2g fiber

Hydrating and delicious, this melon refresher is a light option for heart-conscious individuals.

Cranberry Apple Euphoria

Preparation Time: 10 minutes

Serving: 2

Ingredients:

- ❖ 1 cup cranberries (fresh or frozen)
- ❖ 2 apples, cored.
- ❖ 1 pear, cored.

Instructions:

1. Juice cranberries, apples, and pears.
2. Serve in elegant glasses for an extra touch.

Nutritional Information:

110 calories, 28g carbs, 1g protein, 0.5g fat, 6g fiber

Cranberries are known to support heart health, making this a delightful and beneficial concoction.

Blueberry Basil Bliss

Preparation Time: 12 minutes

Serving: 2

Ingredients:

- ❖ 1 cup blueberries
- ❖ 1 cucumber
- ❖ Fresh basil leaves

Instructions:

1. Juice blueberries, cucumber, and fresh basil.
2. Pour into glasses and enjoy the refreshing blend.

Nutritional Information:

100 calories, 25g carbs, 2g protein, 0.5g fat, 5g fiber

Blueberries, rich in antioxidants, combined with basil, create a blissful and heart-healthy juice option.

MEAL PLANNER JOURNAL

WEEKLY PLANNER

MONDAY	TUESDAY

WEDNESDAY	THURSDAY

FRIDAY	SATUREDAY

SUNDAY	NOTE

WEEKLY PLANNER

MONDAY	TUESDAY

WEDNESDAY	THURSDAY

FRIDAY	SATUREDAY

SUNDAY	NOTE

WEEKLY PLANNER

MONDAY	TUESDAY

WEDNESDAY	THURSDAY

FRIDAY	SATUREDAY

SUNDAY	NOTE

WEEKLY PLANNER

MONDAY	TUESDAY

WEDNESDAY	THURSDAY

FRIDAY	SATUREDAY

SUNDAY	NOTE

WEEKLY PLANNER

MONDAY	TUESDAY

WEDNESDAY	THURSDAY

FRIDAY	SATUREDAY

SUNDAY	NOTE

WEEKLY PLANNER

MONDAY	TUESDAY

WEDNESDAY	THURSDAY

FRIDAY	SATUREDAY

SUNDAY	NOTE

WEEKLY PLANNER

MONDAY	TUESDAY

WEDNESDAY	THURSDAY

FRIDAY	SATUREDAY

SUNDAY	NOTE

WEEKLY PLANNER

MONDAY	TUESDAY

WEDNESDAY	THURSDAY

FRIDAY	SATUREDAY

SUNDAY	NOTE

WEEKLY PLANNER

MONDAY	TUESDAY

WEDNESDAY	THURSDAY

FRIDAY	SATUREDAY

SUNDAY	NOTE

WEEKLY PLANNER

MONDAY

TUESDAY

WEDNESDAY

THURSDAY

FRIDAY

SATUREDAY

SUNDAY

NOTE